Snapshots
of a
Stroke Recovery

Pieter Egriega

PIETER EGRIEGA

This book is dedicated to:

Sareth

My daughters, Phoebe and Ashleigh

My mum Dorothy

All NHS staff, who although they have their failings, saved my failings

The Stroke Association

PIETER EGRIEGA

SNAPSHOTS OF A STROKE RECOVERY

CONTENTS

PIETER EGRIEGA

ACKNOWLEDGMENTS

This book developed out of an original concept given to me that I should create a series of short 100 word stories. It was a brilliant idea, which I grasped enthusiastically. However, in the editing process, I disagreed with the person who provided the original inspiration about the tone that I should adopt in the material. In addition, there was a very real and difficult divergence of opinion about some of the factual components of the book.

I decided that, although I was grateful for the concept, it would be disloyal to other stroke survivors if I railed against the impersonality of medical care and the treatment of the patient as a commodity, and then allowed my writing voice to be amended so radically.

I therefore began rewriting all the stories in a slightly extended format, adding fresh material, as well as one or two stories unconnected directly to my recovery.

PORTRAIT

What I was before June 2013 is irrelevant now. What I was has gone.

I was the co-director of a small software company making smart phone apps. It wasn't particularly successful; it definitely wasn't Microsoft or Facebook or anything, but we had hopes.

I wrote and played bawdy tango songs with a flamenco guitar at folk clubs around the North-West and was banned from quite a few of them. I painted large canvases of women with cat features and I was planning to move on to nudes.

I was large and loud.

That was another person. Some of those things have subsequently continued, but the stroke severed the connection between me and that other person.

This book documents that severance.

SELF – EXPRESSION

The illustrations in this book were done by me, much to my great surprise. Before, I liked to think of myself as an artist, but it was a real effort of will to do these line drawings. Previously I am sure I could have done better. A lot of the character of the sketches has emerged through my inability to hold a pen properly. Even now, I am not particularly comfortable working on drawing and painting as my preferred form of self-expression.

What I am trying to say is that human beings need to express themselves. If I hadn't been able to write or play the guitar, I would have forced myself harder to draw and paint. If I hadn't done any of those, I might have forced myself to cook or to plant vegetables. I would have done anything where I could put effort in and get an output. It is what we do.

Sometimes the world ignores the very best of our work; sometimes the world lauds the very mediocre, but it doesn't stop us. It isn't done to get attention from others, it's done to drive us on...

PIETER EGRIEGA

THE SADIST

It's an incredibly cruel stroke to lose the use of one's fingers during a romantic evening. I'd never slept on this mattress before. I wasn't used to its bizarre memory-foam. To be unbalanced and lose my digital flexibility at the same time, was the work of a sadist.

What was to become of me now? If my right hand wasn't working, there'd be no guitar playing, no ability to paint nudes... did that mean there'd be no more me? Was that it? Was that the end? Bastard!

We called emergency services. The ambulance woman had very little personality, **nor did it seem** any sense of humour. Sareth was calm, though underneath she was frightened by the little she knew. I tried to laugh.

But then I knew nothing.

FOR WHAT DO YOU NEED A SCAN?

Midnight. I am lying in Salford A&E, thanks to Sareth's quick thinking and the relative quiet of Saturday evening roads.

Macclesfield Stroke Ward is closed to new admissions tonight. It feels like they prefer you to be elsewhere if you are seriously ill on Saturday evenings. Government cutbacks I presume or perhaps an exercise in operational efficiency?

In A&E, people look extremely grave at that time of night. Other people's catastrophes are taking place behind flimsy curtains. A trainee doctor from Nigeria looks solemn. He relaxes when I make light of the situation. The principal admissions nurse cheerily asks us difficult questions. She is Indonesian, I think, but she is wonderfully Mancunian in personality.

I'm told I need a CAT scan. Something has been happening in my brain and they need to see what. I am far more concerned with the burgeoning contents of my bladder. There is no need for a scan for that!

CAVES

It is three hours into the situation. I still haven't accepted it's a stroke, although interestingly, I'm on a stroke ward.

I'm not hungry but I am thirsty. My mouth is really dry. I sip some water offered by a male nurse. The water trickles down my throat, like a waterfall into the empty cavern that is my stomach.

I imagine a similar water-filled cave, like the Dragon Cave in Porto Cristo, Mallorca, all stalactites and stalagmites

Then an enormous convulsion shakes me. I am a whale spewing. My body pukes out Jonah. Maybe I'll be all right after this? It is green, watery sludge; there are no carrot chunks. It stinks like the foulest river that ever flowed through any sewer.

Nope, I still can't move my right leg and my right arm.

IT'S WAR

It's dark and I'm in a rubble-strewn room a little like the London Underground in the Second World War. However it feels like I'm in Afghanistan. I can see the night sky in places where there should be roof tiles. Everyone is confused. There are no stars.

I can't hear anything; there's no sound although there should be. At the other end, a gang of soldiers are firing a silent machine gun.

Then a door opens and other soldiers, dressed in the same khaki, roll in a grenade. It explodes. I don't see the shrapnel coming straight towards my head.

I awake in harsh artificial daylight. All the soldiers are still wearing the same uniform. Chaos. They attack each other. Visual explosions shake me but still there's no sound.

I'm on my back, immobile.

TWO MEN

You clot! You bleeding clot! You're a bleeding idiot! That's another fine mess you've got me into.

So here I lie, Laurel and Hardy in one man. The fat one who thinks he's clever. The thin one who's put upon but not as dumb as he's cabbage-looking.

And I'm also two other men: one a moving, throbbing, pulsating man; the other, immobile, a passenger.

You did this you bleeding clot.

It turns out that I had a good heart but I lost my mind.

You're never going to be alone with this schizophrenia.

It's a classic battle. I must find a way to bring my other half back from the dark side.

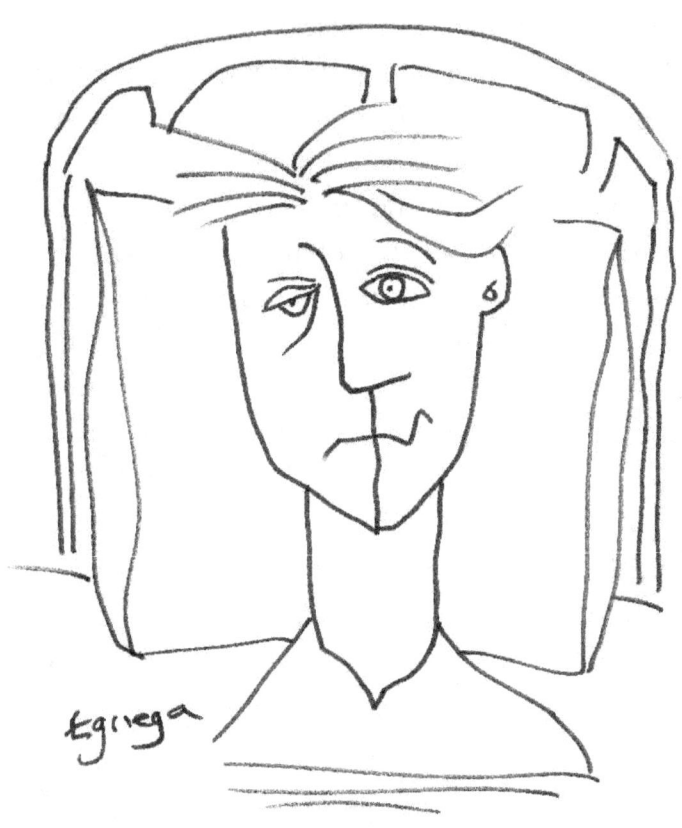

INVENTORY

Two days in. I'm a split physicality.

Left foot: twitching. Right foot: nothing.
Left calf: well formed. Right calf: nowt.
Left thigh: powerful. Right thigh: nil.
Left buttock: thrusting. Right buttock: nada.
Left hand: flexible. Right hand: nichts.
Left forearm: robust and loving. Right forearm: niet.
Left bicep: gun ready. Right bicep: asleep.
Left chest muscle: handsome and pert. Right chest muscle: ugly and slack.
Left eye: bright and uncompromising. Right eye: nonchalant, asleep.

What are these two things doing in the same bed?
I'm separate from myself.

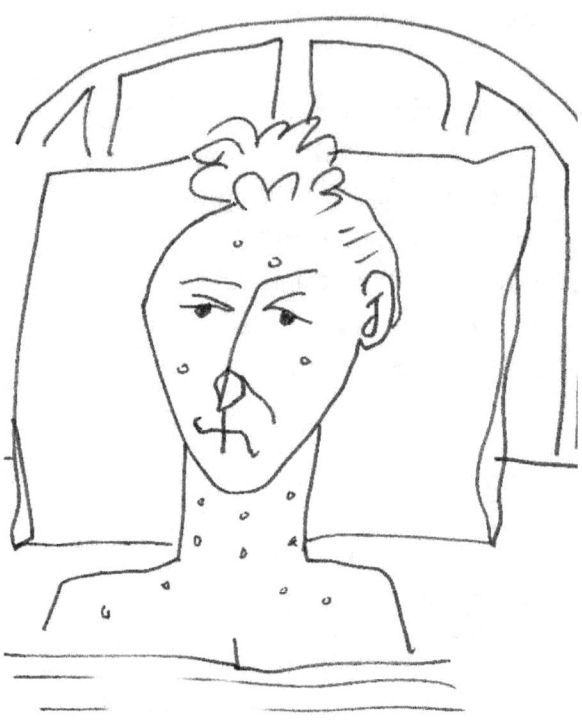

CHICKENS AND TESTICLES

Don't you think that the skin of testicles look like a plucked chicken's neck? If so, that must be why they started talking about their chickens whilst they washed me.

"I've got three," Jane said. "I've got four," said Gail. "I love them to bits."

"Just the two!" I wanted to say... but I wasn't included in their light-hearted chatter.

And they carried on...
"I mix it all up with some of their eggs and a little of their shells."
"Ooh it's uncaring cannibalism," the other said.

"Not really, they haven't had the cockerel."

Unfeeling!

A bit like discussing your chickens over a once proud physique, I thought.

HE'S NOT HIMSELF

Hospital light is harsh and unsympathetic. I see other patients and NHS staff but I'm not connected to anyone. I'm alone.

I'm not myself as I lie in this bed. I can't move. People walk past me, visitors come, doctors conduct interviews about me out of my earshot, nurses discuss their lives.

The enormity of the circumstance dawns on me. Apparently, only 15% of people have my kind of stroke. I could have died, but can I recover?

I determine not to be shy. If this is my destiny, somehow I will embrace my second life and I will tell people about my stroke. Maybe I'll write a book or use my stroke to get known somehow.
Other people become famous for very little, so why not me recovering from this bastard thing?

SELFISH

A relative by proxy through Sareth's family wants to come to visit. As he lives nearby, he has provided a bed to Sareth whilst she visits me. He is 75, and had a debilitating illness 6 months ago and has still not recovered.

I state categorically that I don't want him to come and see me whilst I'm currently more incapacitated than him. The reasons are complex. Male pride in being seen as unhealthy and determination that as I improve it doesn't make him feel worse because his recovery is far slower than mine.

I know, I'm a selfish sod.

IMPORTANT THINGS

It is Tuesday morning. I've hardly slept all night.
I realise that outside, a number of credit card companies, my mortgage, the tax man, my brothers, my business, unhappy clamouring customers, my neglected house, one or two dreams and several ambitions are in the visitors' room pressing for my attention.

They're going to have to wait.

First, I have to stand up. I have to use my fingers. I have to know I can walk again, play the guitar again. I have to hug Sareth and my daughters. Those are the most important things.

Everything else is just incidental.

NO-ONE'S LISTENING

"The patient in 5A. Fifty-five. Male. 19/2/58. Admitted Sunday. Blood pressure controlled by Lisinopril 20mg."
(Hello I'm here!)

"No bowel movement yet."
(Here, over here in the bed!)

"Bottle for urine at night, no need for a catheter. Speech unaffected."
(Here! Behind you!!)

"Right side affected. No mobility."
(Damn it I'm here!!! Can't you see me??)

"Physiotherapy has been alerted. They'll see him from Wednesday."
(Oh for God's sake..!!! Talk to me! Please! Accept and acknowledge my existence... I'm here!!)

"Continue observations. It's a shame for him...
I would hate it if I lost the use of my..."

PERFORMING DOG

I can do nothing. So I do nothing. Somehow boredom is kept at bay. How is it done? Why, through routine of course.

Wake, pee, breakfast, wash, tablets, sheet change, pee, physiotherapy, a gang of doctors, lunch, sleep, pee, visitor, tea, sleep, visitors, pee, tablets, sleep.

In between, I have to think and continually answer bloody questions.

Any pain? Headache.
How bad? Two out of ten.
How many fingers am I holding? Two.
Can you feel that? Yes thank you.
Close your eyes, which leg am I touching? Right, now left. Right and now right again.
Open your eyes, touch your nose with your left hand? With your right hand?

Do I get a reward or anything?

THE BLOB

I am a roll-off roll-on ferry.

"Can you roll towards me dear? That's lovely. Sian's getting a new sheet under you. Now roll towards Sian. Great! She's just pulling the sheet through."
You dare...

"Good boy!"

You cow! Why did you have to say that?
I have more respect for another person.

But it turns out that I am not a person, I am a blob. You can't upset it, it has no feelings and it only hurts if you trap its extremities in the bars of the bed cage or twist its bits.

NO SHIT SINCE SALFORD

The air in hospitals is poisonous. You're less likely to die in a fast food restaurant. Do you want MRSA with that?

We treat everyone the same and everybody is an individual. Yeah right... so how's that gonna work?

Just because I can't move my right hand side, it doesn't make me less capable of outwitting you, doctor, but the doctors are not as bad as some of the nurses.

I haven't shit since Salford!

I'm hoping they'll see that statement for all its alliterative intelligence. But they just thought I was coarse.   My mistake. Maybe I have lost my common sense somewhere? Is that what they call cognitive impairment?

NO INFORMATION

It is late Friday evening in Macclesfield... my blood pressure readings spike and crash in turn. They wheel me out of my cosy private room onto a cardiac ward; surely I can't be having a heart attack as well?

In the corridors, I expect to meet injured Friday night revellers... but no, tonight it's a night of quiet gloom.

I begin to panic, in spite of the pleasantly efficient staff. Do I see panic in the nurses' and orderlies' eyes?

What are they not telling me? What do they know?

Even worse, what don't they know?

CHANGING WARDS

It is Saturday morning in a ward full of women. Not as interesting as you might think. Morag opposite is unsurprisingly Scottish; she is also elderly and belligerent. The nursing staff tread carefully to reduce the possibility of conflict.

The lady to my right is always hidden behind curtains. At visiting time, her relatives want to know where she has hidden the pills and the money. I see a heavily tattooed arm in a wall mirror opposite.

Diagonally opposite, a pleasant fulsome woman in her twenties, a mother, is waiting to be discharged.

By the time I'm moved four days later, it's a ward full of men.

ETERNAL ENTERTAINMENT

Over the ward, the moon hung like a sword.
As we flew round the corner, the rear doors were
open and I nearly fell out.

I woke up with **crowds** of spectators round me.
"One, one thousand, two, one thousand, three,
one thousand."

The nurse who was pounding on my chest said,
"You seem remarkably cool after what just
happened."
I said, "It's okay, there was an invisible man
calming me."

I had no idea who he was.

"We don't need you yet," he said. "You've got
things to do here first.   Now pull yourself
together."

"But who? What? Why? How?" I shouted silently.

He just waved.

TWO TOO MANY

I've got two brothers, Andy the youngest and David the middle brother. I am the eldest in the family, my mother having died last year. Inevitably they visit, possibly worried, amongst other things, about their own mortality.

It's really difficult. Ten days into this physical incapacity, I can't follow one as he paces round the bed, trying to make sense of my circumstance, nor am I able to concentrate on the other brother as he struggles to articulate a thought to me and the other visitors.

I have to ask them both not to come again until I have recovered. It's too difficult for everyone.

STATIC POTENTIAL

He's just lying there. This man, so big even when still. He once appeared to fill the room simply with his presence, his voice, his movements. Now he's been cut down to a blob on a bed by a few bloody brain cells.

I am that blob.

Friends fuss. Nurses notice. Doctors drone. Consultants consider. Physiotherapists pontificate.

So where do we go from here?
It's a slow road. No-one knows how long my recovery will take. No-one knows how complete it will be. No-one tells me anything.

There are so many variables it seems and they know that so much depends on me!

A GOOD SIGN?

It's morning, no-one is around in the ward. Suddenly my right leg goes into a violent spasm. I am surprisingly calm. I let the spasm work through.

I see it is a good sign. It's the muscles in my right leg saying, "Excuse us! We're used to activity and action commands. What's happened? Has someone shot the messenger?"

I'm an optimist. I see this as a sign of potential.

I tell the nurses, the doctors, my visitors, anyone who will listen all about my interpretation of this but no-one confirms that I'm right.
Am I wrong?

The most important thing is to make this arm and leg work again.

WHERE HAS DAD GONE?

I have two daughters, the elder, a step-daughter.
What did they think of me before?
What do they think of me now?
I was probably just the epitome of dad jokes and a
theoretical paternal model.
Now it's changed.
Now I am mortal.
I can't put my right arm round them. I can't hold
them by the hand.
I need to overcome this to show them that some
things in life can be fought.
I need to watch them grow, have children, forge
careers.
I need to be the one they want to make happy
until they find their man.
I must become their hero for the time being.

NURSING SINISTER

The constant change of staff gives me maudlin
thoughts.
No man is an island. Agency staff. I remember the
name Beverley Allitt.
Do poisoners smile when they dispense their
goodies or do they remain terse?
Are they concentrating because it is new to them
or because wicked actions deserve a wicked face?
Most Caribbean women that I had encountered
before were jolly women.
But this new nurse does not even smile?
I develop these sinister thoughts. She could draw
the curtain around any of us and administer what
she wanted. I'm staying awake for as long as I can!

Ah, it's better now! She's talking in that lovely
singsong Trinidadian accent to William opposite.
I'm not worried anymore.

TOUGH ACT

I was big and strong and bright.

I could sketch a face in single lines with no shading.
I could work out a chord sequence from almost all popular tunes and occasionally complex jazz pieces.
I could make up melodies to my own words.
I transposed the keys to most songs whilst I played.
I could analyse form in The Racing Post. I understood the key in the form.
I could do reasonably complex mental arithmetic.
Equally, I could do something quite complex physically, like the butterfly stroke in swimming.

'Now let's see you do something really difficult... Pull your pants up!'

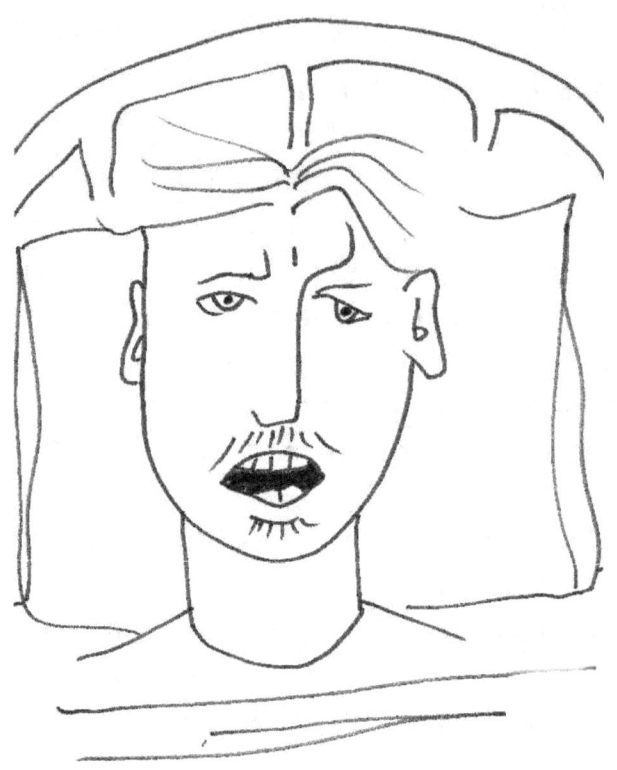

MACHINES ON THE EDGE

We have all these machines to keep the patients going: blood pressure monitors, thermometers, oxygen masks, lights to shine in your eyes, CAT scans, heart monitors, ultrasound scanners. All to keep an eye on these fragile machines... us!

We see robust apparatus in big metal boxes that requires strong men to pull it around. It is connected by thin, coloured wires to pathetic, colourless machines who are now lying exhausted on beds, breathing very shallowly.

These flesh machines once had far greater potential... now they are all contained inside a thin layer of skin, within six foot of flesh, bones, blood, sinews, tendons and damage.

YOUNG AND OLD

This place is filled with the young and the old. The young have no knowledge of life it seems, but are capable of physical acts and medical care well beyond that which the old can now provide.

The old are helpless. They have no life outside of their bodily functions, so they have to have books and light chatter to compensate.

The young make plans for their evenings, their nights, their lives. The old make plans for if they should die... although they can't face that prospect yet.

Where does that leave us? For those who are passive... perhaps it's too late! As for me, I just want to live! I like breathing, I like smelling, I like tasting, I like sensing, I like thinking - I like being alive.

ALL RIGHT JACK

Across from my bed, I have been provided with extras. Actors playing vignettes, tableaux of alternative outcomes.

The local man, outdoor type, stone mason… a seaman's beard, a bulldog chest, an action man stance.
He can go to the bathroom; he can stand on his own; he's all right. However, gradually hospital is wearing him down.
"You've had a mild stroke… slight loss in the right hand side."
His wife chirps in,
"I told you they're not going to let you drive. Let me take care of that suitcase! I'll do that."

And so it goes on. I can see that he likes being looked after. He likes having his family near him at visiting time. He's growing into his role.

BUREAUCRATIC NONSENSE

Another extra is admitted onto this ward, another character. This time he's from the West Midlands. He's arrived after having a funny turn in the cab of his truck. He's salt of the earth.

But he's not happy being here. Unconsciously, he knows the effect it's all going to have on him.
He always has a story. He manages the tales of his life.

"It's like this fella... he had a stroke, got back the feeling in his arm, was working again after a couple of months... but they wouldn't give him his licence back. Not until they were sure. You know they've got to be sure. That's Health and Safety for you. He got it back eventually."

We're all outraged, as if bureaucracy were working in cahoots with this 'stroke' thing.

CONFUSING INSTRUCTIONS

Above my bed are instructions to staff for when I need to get out of bed.

The words 'Two Transfer Swap' indicate that someone must stand with me whilst a 'trained' person moves the bed and puts a chair behind me.

Previously, the other hospital showed me a way that required only one helper... the chair to my strong left side while I manoeuvre round.

Apparently, it's all to do with safety, their worries, possible litigation. What if I were to fall?

I ignore them.

They talk about the dangers of me being over-confident... but in the same breath they admit that having a stroke makes you lose confidence.

Where's the sense or consistency in that?

ALONE

Tonight's visitors have gone.

I remember that 43 years ago, I didn't follow instructions.

I was a frightened 12 year old, alone, outside our house. A freezing cold November night. I was helplessly illuminated by a moon that sneered at me in the shivering night. I was unable to contact anyone. It was in the days before mobile phones... I worried whether I'd ever be able to put things right?

Hours later, my mum walked round the corner, obviously relieved to see me. She wasn't annoyed. We were both happy that I was back on the right track...

Tonight, I am lying in a hospital bed waiting to see if this time I'm going to get back on the right track...

Will things work out well this time?

PAYBACK TIME

I had a stroke because my blood pressure was too high.

So now the nurses wake me to take my pressure every two hours. I don't sleep and can't relax therefore my blood pressure rises. Some nurses let me sleep, acknowledging this contradiction, others wake me.

The band around my left arm tightens as the machine measures. It feels like my veins are being throttled. There are cannulas and bruises in both arms and the tube of the armband presses against the bruises every time the blood pressure is taken. My pressures rise with the pain.

I feel as if I have to bear this torture without complaint because I didn't take the tablets.

DIFFICULTIES

Despair has been admitted to our ward in the bed opposite. I can't stay in the same room.

I've got to get out of here.

A former professor of engineering, but now he's an incontinent mess. The nurses don't know his name for certain... it's 'Mac' on the board above his bed but his wife calls him 'Ross.' However, when reading from his notes it very much depends upon how much the doctors and nurses care to decipher.

He unhooks his tubes, he refuses food, he falls with a splat onto the hospital floor in the night.
Then at 2.30am every night, Despair addresses his god.

YOU'RE IN TROUBLE

Every man is a dribbler. Some are worse than others. A major leak can be hidden in dark clothing. A few droplets are conspicuous on grey trousers.

But with a bottle, you are held hostage by one maverick globule of wee.

I've tried all possible positions and all sorts of techniques. Left side, right side, on your back, the finger wring, the vigorous shake, the foreskin reveal. None of them work. I indulge in five minutes of assorted techniques and then I feel certain there's none left.

But the minute I remove the bottle it emerges, like a golden ambush in my ureter. Pissing hell! A yellow reminder of my lack of control.

DOCTORS AND NURSES

It's the dead of night, the ward is asleep. In the bed opposite, there's a large young man who wasn't there earlier. The nurse is arguing with a young doctor. She won't accept responsibility for this new patient, who has escalating blood pressure, dangerously over 225 from what I can understand.

The young doctor says he'll take responsibility, but she says that after he's gone off duty in an hour, she will still have the worry. She stands her ground. He should be in intensive care. Thankfully, their patient is unconscious.

It seems to me that the doctor is driven by the self-confidence of youth, not experience. She, however, fights for common sense.

Next morning, his bed is empty. But I'm still there and I'm very uneasy that there are confrontations and uncertainties, even in a hospital.

TREATING LAZINESS

I had to apologise to two nurses this morning.

To the first one for previously describing a grimace as my 'fuck face', whilst trying to undertake a simple, but for me, difficult movement of my right leg.

The other one for asking for her help to apply butter and marmalade to toast.

"Do it yourself," she said politely. She was right. Although I was tired, giving in like that is no way to get better. I'd embraced laziness, which had to stop. It is no way to progress.

I need people like her to remind me not to surrender to my innate, human lethargy.

THE COMMUNAL VISIT

Today, I've slaved over my hospital routine,
enjoyed the indifferent catering, Sudoku, a
BBC i-player episode called *What does an Artist do
all day?* and a ruthless physiotherapy session.

I doze off after beef stew and yoghurt for my
evening meal to be confronted... no, shocked... no,
outraged!

Around my bed on assorted chairs, were sitting
seven 50- 60-year old folksingers.

I don't recognise them at first... some take me
more than a few moments to recognise.
It's uncomfortable at first. I'm suspicious.

Why are they here?

I hope, for crying out loud, that they don't sing me
a song with 53 verses!

MADNESS.COM

What happens between the sheets of the hospital stays between the sheets of the hospital.

Old Mr Kyriakos cries out for Kathleen, though his wife is called Reina.

Mrs Baltimore-Rugeley looks through your cupboards looking for her son, her Volvo and her stabled horses.

Delirium for me is now the new normal.

Dana's seen it all and cleaned most of it off the mattress.

Thailand is next door to Burma, we decide, as we discuss where a patient was born.
The bell rings, visitors come and go and Ross wants to die every night at 2.30, as regular as a broken clock.

Yep, that's right. I've seen it all through the bed bars of this Bedlam.

EXPERT WITNESS

In the last few weeks, I've become an authority on many things in which previously I had no interest.

I know about shoulder cuff muscles, triceps, biceps, and pectorals. I can discuss with doctors potassium levels, the correct blood pressure range and the meaning of the two blood pressure readings. I can converse with a dietician about salt levels in processed food. I could, if asked, advise athletes on techniques to improve their performance by visioning, or mental imagery.

What I don't know is how to walk or lift my right arm or avoid that hollow feeling when I realise how far away I am from being normal.

CIRCUIT TRAINING

Yesterday, the two physiotherapist chaps, one either side, helped me stagger up the corridor. This created over-confidence.

"By Friday, I'm gonna walk the ward circuit!" I pronounce.

"Steady on! Set yourself realistic targets," they calm. Deep down, I knew I couldn't have taken a step without them.

Today, another walk. I'm pathetic and unbalanced. We pass yesterday's point and keep going. We move a wheelchair and a hoover aside and continue.

Halfway round the circuit, heading back to my bed, I'm shattered but proud.
But... did we get round this challenge to raise my self-esteem or was it always part of the programme? I don't know.

BOMBER WATSON

He arrives by stealth. "Where am I?" he asks beaming.

"Macclesfield." we say.

He's been parked next to an empty bed in a wheelchair. He doesn't move and he's still there twenty minutes later.

"I don't know who I am."

Sareth looks in his bag. "It says Angus in one bag, but Ian in another."

"That's me, Angus Ian Watson!" he grins. "I flew bombers in the war you know." He smiles.

A squadron of nursing assistants land, draw the curtains and winch him into bed.
"Can we get you anything?"
"Yes, a bottle and a blonde please!"

The chunky matron with peroxide curls looks distinctly uncomfortable as she walks past.

GRANTED IMMUNITY

It's 8pm and most visitors have left.

The ward is quiet. Then, there's activity in our bay. An orderly enters pushing a machine. It's a mobile X-Ray. The nurse politely asks the remaining visitor to leave for five minutes...

The machine is put in place and the operator puts on a leaden apron and ducks under a special canopy, while he positions the X-Ray on the patient in the bed opposite.

The operator asks the nurse to ensure that everyone leaves and closes the door. The other patients can stay.

Doesn't it matter if we're exposed to what everyone else must avoid?

Have our strokes made us immune?

OCCUPATIONAL ADVOCATE

Jacqueline Jackson visits patients and wears a white uniform with green trim. She's discussing the imminent 'home visit' of the chap in the next bed, part of the discharge assessment.

Today, I'm on her list. I complain about being treated like an imbecile by many of the staff. I protest that I'm determined not to surrender to my disability.

She sympathises, then persuades me to join the horrendous breakfast club. She is chatty and I realise she is the first reasonable person here and she acts like an advocate.

She's on the side of stroke survivors by personality, not job role.

You can't interview people for that.

MIXED VISITING

Two friends enter. Both intelligent people, he develops software, she's in funeral care. They sit down, offer cake, discuss the NHS and Syria.

My middle brother, a cheery builder, bashes through the doors and commands a chair.
There's an uneasy silence. My two friends sit stiffly. I'm not really giving them my full attention.

The farce is further enhanced by the arrival of a vicar friend... he's full of activity, dispenses smiles to a terminally ill patient, says a few polite hellos.
He sits down, proclaims something about God's mercy. My brother half-jokingly challenges him.

Everyone looks uncomfortable.

Where do I fit in?

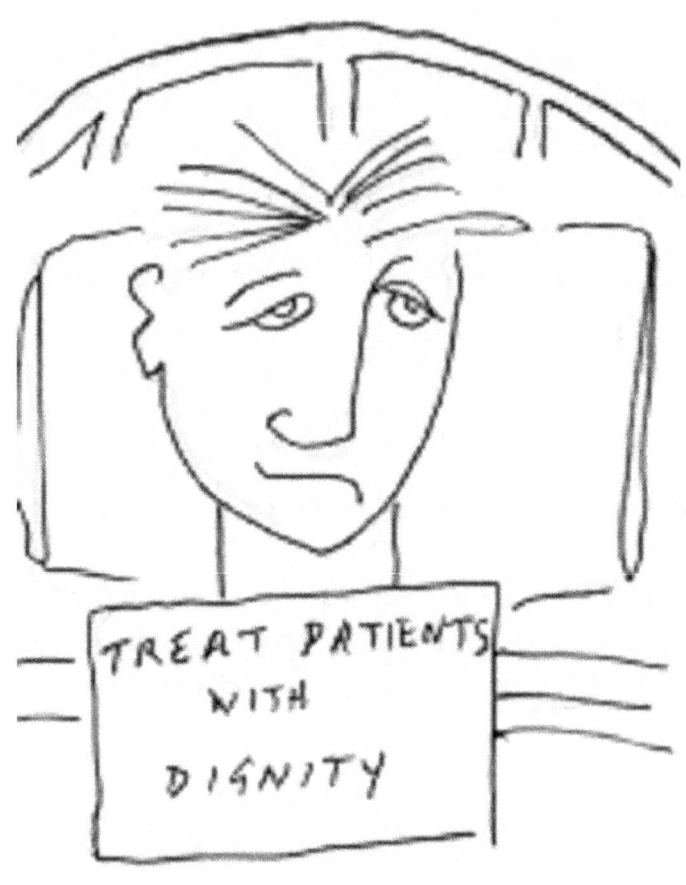

DIGNITY IN HOSPITAL

The nurse is there as I'm waking.

"Good morning, have you moved your bowels?" I imagine that the whole ward is turning their heads with bemused interest in my colonic activity.

Later that day, with help, I remove the sign in the main hospital that says *We Seek to Treat Patients with Dignity.*
I discover two things.
1. Nurses must ensure that your colon and digestion is working... if not... there could be complications.
2. Asking personal questions should, where possible, be done in private.

Next day, there's a different nurse. I'm lying on the bed. The sign is on my chest.

"Any pain? Have you moved your bowels today?"
Then, peering from behind her clipboard.
"PIETER! That sign is hospital property!"

BULLY FOR HIM

Robert Fast is admitted late one evening.

He's 89 and was transferred from a local nursing
home. He's a well-known character here. Has he
had a stroke? Maybe it's the only bed available?
He's a loud Geordie who takes no prisoners.
"There's something about you that I don't like!"
He points to one of the male nurses.
His colleagues smirk.

It seems like Bob's hit a nerve but I never find out
what the other nurses dislike about their
colleague.
Bob has a cuddly toy bull called Chuck. He tells it
everything.
"Well Chucky, this is a right carry on."
"Just you and me now Chuck, we're all that's left."
"Bastards."

DESPERATE TO GO

No-one comes when I press the button. It's been three quarters of an hour (two minutes).

I need to go.
It's started its journey from my bladder.
I rang two hours ago for a bottle (three minutes).

Don't they like me?
Am I worthless because I can't get out of bed?
Shall I wet myself? That'll teach the NHS.
Ah, but then, I'll have to lie in slowly cooling urine... so that's no good.
It's been all day since I had the feeling that I wanted to go. Why doesn't someone come?

"Oh hello. Yes, I just need a bottle. In your own time - whenever you are ready."

THE BREAKFAST CLUB

Two weeks in, I am introduced to 'The Breakfast Club'.

The idea is to get used to real life situations: preparing breakfast, pouring coffee, helping yourself to cornflakes, introducing milk and sugar, buttering toast.

It's stated that they cannot consider discharge of a stroke patient unless he can demonstrate facility in the kitchen! It's a shame for people to be consigned to hospital through a deficiency in domestic ability.

Kevin in the bed next to me avoids going each day, always citing some illness or other.

I wonder why?

What does he know after three months that I don't?

Ah! I see what might be putting Kevin off. Is it perhaps nurses patronising us as they help out?

PHYSIOTERRORISTS

A pathetic, inelegant, shuffling blob made fourteen steps... seven left ones and some silly ridiculous right steps that somehow added up to seven.

Apparently, it is usual to cry at such an achievement on the Stroke Ward but I didn't.
What achievement is there in conquering walking?
I've already done it once before.
Fifty-three years and six months ago. It seemed nothing then.

I've got to set targets.
I set them already on day one. I'm not amending them now on day twenty-four.
Running would be good, climbing would be better!
Then the physiotherapist brings out the step.
"Okay tough guy. Give me ten!"

These physiotherapists, they know what they're doing!

BOXING CLEVER

As a young man I was always quite 'handy'. I wouldn't necessarily take on a muscle-bound night club doorman but if someone were out of order, I wasn't afraid to put them right... physically.

Now I'm a lot less handy.
When the physio says: "Lift your right arm up from the shoulder and point to your nose," I set about myself with a flapping hand that pokes me in the eye, slaps my cheek and I end up with fingers up my nostril.

Not boxing quite so clever now, am I?
Serves me right for being out of order.

SELECTIVE DEAFNESS

At 2.30 in the morning, patients call out.

There is snoring, loud, thunderous rattles. But there are also cries for help, moans, requirements to pee, statements of their pain, bottom burps.

But it's no laughing matter. Nearest to me, Ross had a stroke, he has liver cancer and pneumonia. After falling out of bed, pulling out the feeding tubes and loudly voiding his bowel, he calls for his god to release him.

Throughout the day with his wife by the bedside, he sleeps or makes incomprehensible noises.

But there's something about the early hours that brings out the dark thoughts and the demons.

I have to ring because the nurses don't always seem to hear his bell constantly ringing.

UNHAPPY

The physiotherapists suggest that soon we can talk about going home.

I apply myself to their exercises. We do the usual half hour. I enjoy doing it because I am challenged and treated like an adult.

Exercised to their satisfaction, I need the toilet.
I use the wheelchair; I'm not confident walking unaided. I tell the patient opposite where I'm going.

Immediately inside the bathroom, I hear commotion outside. I lock the door and pull across the curtain.

I find out that I have done wrong. As a result of needing my privacy, I've upset the nurses who are frightened because their procedures have been violated. They fear I may collapse and come to more harm.

A STATE OF MIND

Kay the physiotherapist says, "Today I'd like to see how you do a car transfer."

I am pushed outside in a wheelchair. The air is different. I transfer my bottom first and easily swivel my legs into the car. Phew! It would seem that there'll be no problem... when it's time to leave hospital.

"Right, why don't you two have a little drive? See you in an hour."

I look at her without understanding. Sareth is already in the driver's seat.

We drive through the car park. "You look worried," she says.

It's true, I am terrified!

Do I want to escape? What am I leaving, a stroke ward or an institutionalised state of mind?

TIRED VISITING

When one person suffers a stroke, others are directly affected. My work colleague discovers I can do nothing to help him. My romantic companion of only one year discovers that her life has been devastated.

At first, she tries to visit me three times a day. The afternoon and evening visiting, as well the morning cleaning ritual. It's too much for her, even after she discovers she can park in staff parking next to the stroke ward doors.
She is absolutely worn out.

She agrees she will wash my undercarriage in the morning and then visit in the evening only.

Meanwhile, I lie in bed like royalty. An immobile privileged pee-r.

IT'S PERSONAL

The question of personal hygiene is, well, personal.

Where there's no control, one can understand the need for a community to take action over the individual, the mad, the bad and the sad... but why does a stroke suddenly turn me into a freak that needs to be accompanied on every bathroom visit?

What unique pleasure do certain nursing staff derive from wiping my bottom and generally giving me the once over with a flannel?

Why the same question every morning, asking if I need help showering?

Had I realised that I was capable of generating such interest in middle-aged women, my recent sex life might have been considerably more enjoyable.

COMMITTEE CONFUSION

Occupational Therapy are talking about me going home for a short stay, but they can't decide if it is for a night or a weekend.

Not only can they not agree, but doctors and nursing staff must have their say. Like all decisions by committee, they can't concur, so there is no decision.

They want to design a holiday for me but they are actually extending my prison sentence!

Eventually at 6.55pm, we're told we can perhaps stay at home tonight but we are given different times for returning.

Brilliant!

We will use their lack of clarity to do exactly what we want!

USE THE STUPID STICK!

There are bigger arseholes than me but I have my days. Today was one such day.

I'm walking outside my bay with the lady physio at my side. Previously, we discussed that the problem with using a stick is that it might make me too reliant.

Today, she gives me a stick to aid my balance on this the third day of walking.

In my head I'm thinking, "Don't use the stick."
I lift the stick up, carry it like a spear.

She's furious because she was assessing my competence for walking safely before I can be discharged. Now she has to say that I'm not safe yet!

I am, without doubt, a first class pillock!

COGNITIVE ASSESSMENT

Today is cognitive assessment day.

I've heard the test twice before on two different wards in two different hospitals. Here she comes, reading her clipboard, she walks towards me.

I don't say anything, it's not my place. First, I draw clocks; I show her what ten to two looks like and then twenty past four.

Next we discuss the similarity between a bicycle and an aeroplane and between an orange and a banana.

"Now," she says, "I'm going to ask you to remember a list of five words. I will ask you to repeat them back now and then again at the end of the test."

I said, "Will they be FACE, VELVET, RED, CHURCH, and DAISY?"

She looks confused.

"It was just a guess," I confess.

"I'll tell you what, can you think of five different ones?"

"No!" she said.

Who exactly should be cognitively assessed here?

THE FIRST HOME VISIT

It is the morning after the first night home visit. I wake after 10 hours of refreshing, uninterrupted sleep.

The differences between stroke ward life and home are many. The room temperature is cooler than on the ward, yet strangely, it feels warmer inside the sheets.

In the hospital ward, sadly, no-one lies in bed with me. (I'm not counting Mrs Rugeley-Carruthers, who occasionally climbed into my hospital bed, believing she was on the sofa with her dog, Bunbury, watching Channel 4 racing from Ascot.)

At home there's Sareth.

Most notably, I'm not woken by the crash and bang of domestic hospital staff offering morning coffee. Here, there's a warm body breathing gently next to me and a summer morning busying itself in the road, the hedgerows and the fields outside.

HOSPITAL TENNIS

It's Wimbledon women's singles final, the day after my overnight home-visit.

I was expected back earlier but came back after the tennis.

In the ward I look at the other patients. I have to escape.

The nurse is annoyed because I didn't come back earlier. She says she won't discharge me.

Deuce.

We request a doctor, who arrives and says I can discharge myself...

Advantage patient.

... as soon as the ward sister completes the paperwork.

Deuce.

The sister, who doesn't know me, says I can leave but she won't authorise tablets to regulate my blood pressure.

Advantage sister.

I'll have to wait till Monday.

Game, set and match.

She wins, I have to stay.

LACK OF BALANCE

Today I shouted at a nurse. I lost my control. Just like I lost control of half of my body.
Tired of the constant patronising, I could take no more and I let rip.

The simpering voice, "Want me to take you for a little wash and then you can open your bowels?"

"No, I want you to treat me with the bit of dignity that I think I deserve! I wouldn't undress in front of you normally, so you're not getting your 'better than you' kicks today! Sod off!"

Affronted, she just stared at me demanding some kind of emotional balance.

My apology was not forthcoming.

It seems that I'm not a gentleman.

GOOD NEWS

I see someone who looks familiar, walking through my ward. At exactly the same minute, there's recognition.

"Oh my God, how long have you been in here?
What are you doing here? Yeah, I work on different wards, but I haven't been on duty for weeks. We've been on holiday. You know Al had a stroke 20 years ago?"

"Al, guitarist, singer and thoroughly good chap?"
"Yes, but he doesn't tell anyone."
"Was he like me? No right side movement?"
"I don't know, it was before we met."

It was the best thing I'd heard since I had been admitted. If someone can recover and no-one knows, that is great news.

ESCAPE, LIES AND TENNIS

After blocking my escape, they change my bay. I'm in with a younger, less terminally ill, but no less snoring group.

Sareth arrives. I've dressed myself already.
"Let's go!" I plead.

We drive home after telling the nurse in charge that we were going to the restaurant and then would be watching the men's final. We do watch the Wimbledon men's final, but at home. Afterwards, we return to hospital. We chat with nurses in the day room about Andy Murray's victory.

The senior nurse says "We couldn't find you."
"I was in the restaurant." I lie.

Sareth waves goodbye. She has friends coming tonight.

I stay in the day room watching rubbish on the TV.

THE BROKEN MIRROR

I'm to be released. People go away to get medicines and forms. I need the loo. There's no-one around. Previously, I have been chastised for locking the door. Health and Safety, I presume.

I draw the curtain, which is some 10 feet away from the porcelain and start my straining.
The door opens, the curtain moves.

"Anyone in?" It is the young male nurse.
"I'm on the loo," I say with the customary raising of pitch at the end of the statement, as young people do.
"Won't be long, just replacing the mirror... it's broken."

So is any respect for a patient's dignity, I think.

GOODBYE

It's Monday lunchtime.

In the day room, the wife of a terminally ill patient comes in and breaks down sobbing. For the last ten days, I have watched her and her husband's pain. I look down at the floor, as she expresses her despair.
She dries her eyes and asks how I am, then wishes me well when I tell her I am to be discharged.

Afterwards, I'm given a plastic bag filled with medicines and the form signed by the doctor, the ward sister and the physiotherapy team.
I can go.

I get in the car. My recovery really starts now.

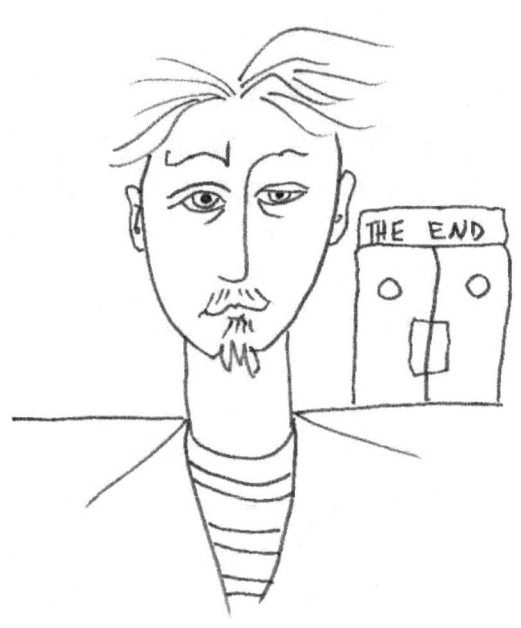

I KNOW SO LITTLE

I've been out of hospital for six days.

Since coming home, Sareth and I walk up the road every day. It's a 100 yards round trip.

Now, I'm ready to take another challenge.
Around the block is barely a quarter of a mile of unsteady terrain. My younger brother comes with me.   Halfway round, the enormity of the task dawns. Walking requires thinking.

Every single step has to be thought through. I need to stagger every other step to help save the weight on my weak leg. Every muscle, every movement needs consideration. How do I do it properly? I don't even consciously know the muscle movements.

No wonder I'm knackered.

SHIP OF DREAMS

I dream about being in a black and white film with lots of establishment shots of a big warship called 'Thessme.' The captain is screaming,
"Get the engine going... more fuel!"

Down in the engine room, the chief engineer is trying to get the ship moving. They are shovelling coal into the boiler. A mechanic is frantically joining pipes.

Up in the ship's bridge, Sareth is looking wonderfully calm, discussing what life would be like when the ship finally gets moving and reaches dry land.

I dissolve and merge into the captain who has lustful designs on Sareth, the leading lady.

What does it all mean?

A DIFFERENT KIND OF EXERCISE

Rehabilitation works. Physiotherapy works, visualising opening the neural pathways works... but you know, you need other stuff too.
Sareth says, "Come with me."

"Why, where are we going?"

"To the supermarket."

"Okay," I say happily. I thought we'd been all over since my release. Wrong again.

Against Sareth's advice, I walk into the sports shop next door to the supermarket. I can feel the eyes of the super-fit staff watching, as I stagger through.
"I'll go and look at exercise bikes." I think.
 No-one approaches me; no-one asks me if I need help.
They all think I must be 'special'.

MY REAPPEARANCE

One week after I leave hospital, there's a folk club night in our village. I push a borrowed wheelchair to the front. I sit in the wheelchair. Everything else is the same. People look over at my disability, some know, some don't.

Then it's my turn to play. I've practised songs. I can manage one guitar strum per bar. My voice soars over the simple arrangement. It feels good. When I have finished, I stagger from the performance area. There's applause. Two singers, unused to commenting on other performers come over. They say I sound better. It appears as if the emotion in my songs is now heard along with the lyrics.

After my stroke, this is the first thing that is better than before.

THE LITTLE BROWN DEPOSIT

Tonight, I took the dog for a walk. It was a minor task, but to me another milestone on the road to recovery.

I wouldn't win any prizes for elegance or any road safety accolades either but I got around the block without serious injury to me or the dog. I can't guarantee that she didn't defecate on anyone's garden but I'm hoping a sense of neighbourly charity will cover up that little mess.

Perhaps the sight of me being dragged along will assist to erase the sight of the little brown turd lurking in the centre of that neatly manicured lawn?

FRANZ KAFKA'S BADGE

We apply for disabled blue badge status.

I receive a letter. I must go in person to the library, which is 200 yards from the car park, although it's only 10 yards from the three disabled parking spaces. However, I can't use them: I haven't got a badge.

Sareth drops me at the library door, car horns honk as I annoy other drivers, because I'm struggling to get out of the car. I stumble and stagger to the library reception. Obviously, it is part of the deal - they have to make it difficult to get a badge.

Perhaps the authorities would prefer it if I were in a wheelchair?

INTERCONNECTIONS

When I was young, I was always intrigued by kaleidoscopes. I know they were just a series of mirrors and bright, shiny, glass beads. The attractive quality came about as you turned the tube and saw all the working parts interlocking.

So it is with our lives; we are all interconnected. Except I remember the cheap children's toy of the 1960s, containing discoloured rogue beads which didn't fit properly. When your kaleidoscope is a testament to rough play, frequently something will go wrong. If the whole isn't working correctly, it isn't interlocking, it won't interconnect.

So it is with my life... until I can get better.

BATH TIME FOR JONAH

I've been poorly all day. I'd overdone it the day before.

By 8pm, I fancy a bath not a shower. We take the view... if I can get in, I can get out.

It's wonderful to rest my aching body in the warm water (helpful, as I was encrusted in bits of vomit and poo), but after I let the water out, I realise how horribly wrong I can be. I am stuck.

Barry the handyman hasn't as yet put a rail on the bathroom wall. The adhesive qualities of my arse will go down in the annals.

Call the fire brigade........ there is a beached whale!

MOWED DOWN

It is a warm summer's day in late July six weeks after my stroke. The previous weeks have seen a lot of growth in our garden. Sareth is going out for the day and I hatch a plan to mow the lawn whilst she is out, to surprise her.

The lawn has three areas, a large main section about 20 feet by 10 feet and two secondary areas, each about 10 feet by 10 feet. In terms of achieving something, it is a good idea. In terms of my fatigue... BIG MISTAKE.

I set off full of grand ideas and good intentions, dragging my right leg around the lawn and lifting the 25lb hover mower but mostly with my left hand. I get through one length of the main lawn and am ready for several hours sleep. Somehow, almost nauseous with exhaustion, I finish the main area and decide that for all my ambition, the other two lawns can wait. I put away the mower and leave the cuttings in the bin in the centre of the lawn. Desperately, I get in the house, fall onto the sofa in the living room and within seconds, I'm asleep.

Sareth wakes me several hours later with a kiss and the words, "You bloody silly sod."
I haven't the energy to smile but I'm extremely happy.

STROKE GYM

I am persuaded to go to the Stroke Survivors' Gym at the local leisure centre. It is a shock. I meet survivors with a wide range of ongoing disabilities.
I'm smug.
It is misplaced.

My walking is appalling but a few of the others are worse.

By the end of the hour, I have cried, I have sweated, I have grimaced, I have given up and I have gritted my teeth and continued.

When the exercise leader shouts, "Raise your hand high!" I gloat and lift my good hand better than anyone.

When she says, "And now the other arm!" I try to lift my bad arm...

I'm actually worse than the worst of them.

CEILIDH AND THE REST

It is mid-August. We've been invited to Scotland to Amy Geddes' birthday celebrations.

We're assigned a beautiful little barn conversion owned by a doctor.

It's calm and peaceful.

I sleep off and on for one third of the weekend.

I play the guitar after the four-hour drive and I sing gently.

Sharon the doctor slips into the room and asks about my recovery. She tells us that musicians have a good chance of getting the neural pathways in the brain to fire again. She says she's seen some research that suggests there are all sorts of ways that this happens.

I pretend I understand, but I don't care; it's all fantastically good news.

BOYS AND THEIR PILLS

Most people don't know much about strokes until they have one.

Everyone knows about smoking, obesity, lack of exercise. My stroke was caused by high blood pressure. As both my brothers know, it's hereditary.

I stopped taking blood pressure tablets about two years before my stroke because my GP mentioned that one of the tablets might affect sexual performance.

We can't have that now can we?

We'd rather have no movement, be treated like an inanimate blob by all concerned, unable to do everything we did before, have our partner fill in forms and wipe our arses, than have our sexual performance affected... hey boys?

CRIPPLED WITH KINDNESS

I phone a business associate, who is well aware that I've had a stroke.

"And how are you?" I ask.

"I'm a cripple today," he replies, without a trace of irony. "I bruised my foot in the garden yesterday."

I hear him register that his initial statement was insensitive and inappropriate but he's the type who very rarely apologises for a faux pas. He would see it as a sign of weakness in his personality.

"Oh, that makes two. We can hobble in sympathy."

I'm conscious that our combined disability doesn't really warrant the emotive word 'cripple!'

How kind am I?

THE INK BLOT

Today I am an ugly blot, an asymmetrical ink splodge.

Rorschach would have a field day assessing my walk. That's if you accept the idea that we are what we look like.

But who made my imperfection? Well I did! Although not intentionally, I arrogantly avoided medical advice.

Why? Perhaps just so that I could be different? Well I got that sub-conscious wish.

Now, I'm too different for lorry drivers and builders. Different from the sporty, different from the aggressively, acquisitive. Different, yet apparently ordinary.

I want your sympathy... but I'd hate to get it.
Go on, analyse that one if you can!

THE TIME WARP

I go back in time 93 days. It's an early June Saturday evening. We decide to take a picnic into the park in Knutsford prior to watching a French film in the Curzon Cinema.

I remember sprinting back to the car to find the bottle opener.

It is a lovely picnic, olives, ham, chutneys, flatbreads and a dark red wine. Other people look on enviously. Another family behind us are preparing a communal curry. A small flotilla of geese land ceremoniously on the reservoir.

It's been a busy day.

Five hours later I am lying in A&E having lost it all.

THE EQUILIBRIUM OF DREAMS

I read somewhere that pop stars, politicians and international athletes have fairly mundane, pedestrian dreams, whereas petrol pump attendants, local government officers and bin men have exotic fantasies whilst sleeping. It's the collective unconscious undertaking a kind of balancing act.

Whilst in hospital, I rarely slept deeply enough to be able to remember any dreams and the first two nights home provided such refreshing sleep that I forgot any dreams.

But since then whoa..............!
I've chased leopards through the streets of London, fought a voodoo octopus in the seas around Formentor in Majorca and generally been rampant in a fashion show where all models look like Sareth.

Maybe it's just me?

AND A SPECIAL THANKS

Imagine a world where you have no control.
It's not that hard to do.

Imagine all the people and only a few of them come to help.

Sareth has been my life since my stroke... kept me going, cheered me up, talked about possibilities, took care of the mundane things.
It's difficult to brush aside the thoughts that darken someone's mind and get them to focus on what they have 'now!'

If you are reading this because you've had a stroke, I hope you have loved ones in your life.
If you are The One in someone's stroke, thank you!

SENSE & SENSUALITY

I have an appointment with a lady from the Stroke Association.

First we discuss my stroke, then anonymously, other people's strokes, weight loss, diets and whether I can claim benefit. We don't think the system will help me out.

It's a nice day. We laugh a little about all sorts of things. Then at the end she turns somewhat serious.

She isn't embarrassed but clearly she wants to introduce a delicate subject.

She says discreetly, "For many people, there is the question of sex after a stroke."

Just then Sareth enters the room and says,
"No problem. What is it that you want to know?"

CONSIDER THIS

Everyone who knows about strokes says it's the loss of control that has the most debilitating effect. They don't mean control of legs, arms, hands, temper, and desire.

So if you don't know… think that one through.
To lose your motor functions, your drive to 'do', is not as bad as the 'other lack of control'. They actually mean control over 'your life'.

If you are tempted to ask a stroke survivor,
"Need help washing yourself?" or you ask a stroke survivor's companion, whether 'he' wants something?

STOP!
REWIND!

Please ask yourself:
How would you feel if someone said that to you?

SCARY FLESH

In the first week of hospitalisation, I experienced spasms in my arm and leg. Far from being scared by involuntary muscle movements, I was comforted because I thought my muscles were complaining that they'd had nothing to do.

Today the physiotherapists finally injected some medical common sense into it. It's the muscles switching on.

The other night I had a scare. My calf muscle went into spasm. I lifted my leg, stood firmly on the floor only to find that my calf had contracted very tightly and the flesh was so loose that it hung from the muscle... funny really, it wasn't even Halloween yet!

BENEFIT NUMBER TWO

Has someone left the tap on in the house, because the water pressures are down? Is it Pieter? In the days before the stroke, I'd previously left the gas on, the hot water on, the lights on and the toilet seat up. I hear them discussing me.

They run upstairs. No, they confirm, the water is turned off.

They agree that I now turn the lights off, I don't leave water running and I don't leave the seat up. "That's probably because he no longer pees standing up."

Little do they know. The truth is, I can no longer think beyond what I'm doing. So almost everything is done thoroughly.

I've found number two in a series of benefits of a stroke.

FOETAL EMOTION

In stroke literature, there's a paragraph, stating that stroke survivors can experience very strong emotional responses.

I'm asleep. It's a very vivid dream. Turquoise light suggests I am under water and there's blue coloured vegetation.

In the distance there is activity. A shape emerges. It's my mum, who died last year. She smiles and waves at me just like I remember... I try to tell her everything that has happened but before I can get anything out, she merges into the surroundings again. I wake up in bed, curled up on my left side, covered by blankets.

I cry uncontrollably for several minutes.

BENEFIT NUMBER THREE

Previously, I carried weight well, nearly 18 stone.

Carrying that much weight contributed to my stroke, along with the high blood pressure, which is genetic in my family.

After the first week in hospital, I was one stone lighter because I couldn't eat.
Gradually, I've lost 2 further stone. I avoid 'weighty' foods. No cakes, crisps or petrol station sandwiches for me. Now I fit into suits never before worn, and choose clothes for a much slimmer me. The scales show reductions every week, no salt or sugar, I'm slimmer and healthier.
I look more interesting.

It's the third in a series of benefits of a stroke.

RIGHTEOUS INDIGNATION

The blue badge finally arrives.

We drive to town to watch another French film. There are crowds of boozed-up Mancunians swarming, yet we park next to the cinema door in the centre of Manchester on a Saturday night.

Number 4 in a series of benefits of having a stroke. But there's more.

Next day, as the official badge holder, I go with Sareth to the supermarket.

All the disabled spaces are taken. I stay in the car, as a variety of vehicles use the disabled spaces, with no obvious disabled person or blue badge. I get the chance to feel righteously indignant. Come on... everyone loves a bit of righteous indignation.

MISHEARD SECONDS

Last night we had a homemade chorizo and butternut squash risotto.

To assist my rehabilitation, Sareth says, "If you want more, you should help yourself with your right hand."

I should tell you that it's very difficult to scoop the food out of the pan with a right arm that doesn't work properly, but it was lovely food.

Then today, at my weekly physiotherapy session, Sareth says to the physiotherapists, "Rest assured, I tell him that if he wants seconds he must use his right hand."

The look of shock on the physio and occupational health lady's faces suggest that they have misheard. "And in the end he came back four times."

Then it dawns on us all...

"We are talking about seconds... not sex!"

THE STUPIDITY OF BANKS

Institutions are stupid in the face of a stroke.

"If you could just ask Pieter to sign the form to say you are his representative."

"Err... did we mention that the stroke has left him unable to use a pen? He's right-handed. If he signs with his left hand it wouldn't be the signature you have on file. He can barely use his right hand. I could sign it for him but will you accept that?"

"As long as he sends us a letter to say that he can't write."

"A typewritten letter?"

"Yes, perfectly acceptable!"

"May I type it for him?"

"Yes, okay and if you could just get him to sign it?"

BLACK DOG

Five months into my recovery, I have a very black day: tired, grumpy, emotional, close to giving up and laying down... eyes tired, back tired, I'm exhausted.

I have to be positive, but I can't remain positive all the time.

Sometimes you've got to suck in the blackness. You must accept it or it will destroy you.

I haven't got the strength to remain positive in the face of all the crap... money, limited movement, bills, my problems, other people's problems. I know that I can't solve everything.

They say that what doesn't kill you makes you stronger... but do you know what? At the moment it feels like a very close thing.

SYMPATHETIC AUDIENCE

"Come and address our Regional Conference at Haydock Park," said the Operational Head of the North West Stroke Association.

I agreed willingly. After all, I'm not shy.

One hundred employees of the Association, mostly women of a certain age, filled the large room. "Ooh," said Sareth, "your ideal audience."

We listened to local issues and ideas about best practice fundraising within the region. Then I was up. I recited what I thought was one of my less entertaining stories. The audience spontaneously applauded.

I turned and smiled happily at Sareth. The audience was enjoying it. They laughed at the other stories. I finished off with a song. Afterwards, one by one, members of the audience came to congratulate me.

It was a wonderful feeling to be appreciated. But I guess they knew what I had been through.

WHERE WOULD I BE?

How does anyone cope after a stroke, especially if they don't have someone fighting for them?

Would a friend have wiped my backside?

Would my daughter have been able to ring the benefits agency or the bank?

Who would have assured hospital I could be discharged? Who would have got the safety rails on the stairs? Who would have prepared food other than toast and cereal? Who would have kept my spirits up when I was angry with myself for not walking? Who would have been able to chart my progress upwards?

Where would I be without someone like Sareth?

THE LAND TIME REMEMBERS

Old age is a land you barely perceive and rarely think about. There is a mist around it. I imagine it as a white and grey landscape, flat yet wrinkled. People go there and never come back. They change but don't notice it themselves. You can't get there early if you don't want to go. But eventually you have to go.

But after my stroke I have changed.

I've been dragged close to the border between middle age and old age and yet I'm still too young to be called old by old people.

But scarily, I'm now too old ever to be called young again.

MAN'S BEST FRIEND

The response from the dog has been fascinating.

When I first moved in with Sareth, the dog, Elsie, liked me, partly because we took long walks.

Whilst in the hospital, Sareth and her daughter brought Elsie to visit me. From the car, she was wagging her tail. I was in a wheelchair. When she was released, she came hesitantly, then happily sat on my knee.

Once home and trying to walk regularly, I start taking her with me on the lead.

There's no pulling, she licks my right hand; she seems to know it is the affected side.

Elsie is no dumb animal.

LOCAL TREATMENT

We're invited to have the 'flu jab, at our local medical centre, me because of my stroke and Sareth because she has asthma. We stick out like sore thumbs against a mixture of beige and grey polyester.

I'm tired through a lack of sleep and I'm irritated at being invited to join people who are clearly 20 years older than me.

I stagger into the consultation room and sit down. A middle-aged man, who's spent too long on the sunbed, leans over me, as he would to a mentally deficient geriatric and says, "And how are you today?"

He is very nearly kicked into early retirement!

WHO KNOWS BEST?

A week after I was discharged from hospital, I sat on a bicycle, trying to visualise riding before I set off down the road. I couldn't envision it. I didn't know whether I could ride.

There were two people with me. They dissuaded me from trying. They said I might fall off and I wouldn't be able to stop myself if I started falling.

I sat there for several minutes and then dismounted.

I haven't driven a car in six months either. I don't know whether I can drive...

A doctor and an insurance company have to approve me before I try.

UPS AND DOWNS

I am improved enormously. I can open the fridge door with my right hand. Downside: now I have more access to food that I must resist.

I can walk two miles in a very inelegant way. Downside: I'm teaching my legs bad tricks. However, my stamina is much improved.

I can almost lift my arm up to the top of the door. Upside: I can put my arms round Sareth whilst lying down.

I can write my name. Downside: it's not my signature.

But let's see the positive. For what it's worth, I could forge a drunken, disabled, homeless man's signature!

TAKE IT AWAY

A stroke leaves you powerless.

We're selling my house, so I'll own no house. I have no money. I cannot help my business partner solve problems. I cannot pull my own weight. Stacking the dishwasher or running the Hoover exhausts me. I can provide no material assistance for my daughter. I can't do a proper job.

I'm beholden to my lover. This makes things difficult.

Tonight, she chastises me about opening the car door whilst she is reversing. I rebel and snipe back, without thinking. I'm fed up of my inability. I'm fed up of having to rely on her to fill in forms about my disability. It's horrible being useless.

But what else can I do?

FLORENCE

Florence the Spaniel, who lives near me, was run over a year ago and initially lost the use of her back legs. I would see her dragging her back legs behind her, before I was hospitalised.

Today, whilst we are out, we meet Florence and her owner, trying to improve the walking ability. Florence has more strength in her back legs than before, thanks, we are told, to electronic muscle stimulation. Sometimes, she almost walks normally.

The parallels between us are mentioned, as I try to keep up.

Florence's back legs occasionally collapse under her, whilst mine are totally inelegant.

But I think to myself, if a spaniel can get better, then so can I.

POLITICAL EFFECTS

You know a country by the way it takes care of its people.

I don't know about shirkers, benefit cheats, the work shy, immigrants.

What I do know is that five months after a stroke, inevitably my business is folding; I don't appear to be entitled to receive money from the state because I have been running a business...

I can't demand money from the government to exist... but it would be nice. The problem is there is no safety net.

There's just the haves and the have-nots and then little old me being Bolshie with everyone and not wanting to give up.

THE PROBLEM IS...

In the corporate culture I inhabited, senior management would trot out the aphorism,
"Bring me solutions not problems."
My suspicion was that they were abdicating their responsibility for leadership.

In my little app software business, my co-director's favourite phrase is
"The problem is..."
He likes to demonstrate that our technology is always complex and that for every solution, it's always the case that little problems will creep in.
Of course, both these scenarios bear comparison with my stroke.

I want to get better, so there's no point complaining about the difficulties... I've just got to get on with it.
Secondly, my recovery brings with it unexpected outcomes, some positive, some not.

SURVIVORS

I am being asked to present to groups of stroke survivors and volunteers, as well as other groups.
I'm nervous. My story is my story and however bad my stroke has been, maybe I was lucky and others have been far worse affected? What if other survivors think I'm a fraud because their challenges are far greater than my own? The Stroke Association suggest that I tell my story and allow others to draw their own conclusion and inspiration from it.

I meet at one group, a guitar player called Tony, who befriends me on Facebook and tells me he's playing the guitar again. But then I meet another man, who when I suggest he could make a small step towards his objective tells me that he 'has' to do exactly what he did before. If he can't get that back, there is no sense in trying.

I begin to think that possibly some survivors feel the effect of their stroke so intensely, that they reluctantly accept their disability because they haven't enough energy left to find a way round it.

But no-one should accept their lot, they should try and overcome if they can.

RESISTANCE

Were you as a child enchanted by the idea of resistance fighters battling oppression? I was.

I thought that if the Nazis had invaded and subjugated England when I was a teenager, I would have wanted to bomb military installations and undertaken all sorts of guerrilla warfare, under the cloak of darkness or even in full daylight if I could escape. I'm sure that most people believe there is something noble about fighting an oppressor in such circumstances and possibly like to feel that they could be heroes, either by helping to win the war or at least by contributing to the ongoing battle.

And yet, here we are, one million plus people, affected by stroke every year, oppressed into victimhood, staggering about, clenching our affected side, dragging our bodies through life, assuming that people are going to help us.

I realised that my stroke was my chance to fight back, to bomb the ideology that a stroke survivor is a victim, to incite myself and others into resistance fighting, to overcome and throw off the oppressor.

I might not win a Victoria Cross or the Resistance Medal, or whatever bit of brass they give freedom fighters these days... but this is my chance to break free of stroke's tyranny.

KICKING STROKE'S ARSE

When I had a stroke, my brain lost an area of its ability. That area controlled things: my walk, my arm, my hand. The muscles in those areas didn't stop working, but the brain's tried and tested way of telling my muscles to work had died.

I was lucky. My nerves were still working so I could feel my limbs, but the messages weren't being sent out.

At any time of life, the brain can be trained to do a new thing, such as juggle, ride a unicycle, learn a new language or play a new musical instrument.

You can train your brain to work again if you have had a stroke.

I start by hitching my leg up to walk, as many of us do.

As I write this, my leg does move forward automatically, but it's inelegant. I have to tell my brain to take over all the component parts of my walk. "Heel down, propel momentum through the toes." And so it goes on.

If I keep doing it, my brain eventually gets the idea.

Then I can stop thinking about it.

It's definitely not easy. But why shouldn't I get it all back?

THE BEGINNING

My stroke was an end and a beginning. It was a line drawn under my life up to that point and a chance for reinvention.

This really is my second life. Every day I do things to demonstrate the brand new me.

I am calmer, less stressed, I've lost weight. I have a new focus and I'm grateful for the little things.

You know storytellers always want to blabber on about beginning at the beginning. This is my chance to start again and I'm a contrary sod, so I'm starting at the end. It's not what I would have chosen.

But when reality bites you on the arse AND flips you 180 degrees, what are you going to do? You've got to fight haven't you? You never know; you might just surprise yourself... and all the other buggers.

PIETER EGRIEGA

PANORAMIC VIEWS

A QUESTION OF LOVE

I'm in a pub down a side street in town. I've come in here because I don't want to run into anyone I know.

I sit down with a drink and immediately a 'character' slides along the bench seat from the other end, surprisingly bringing a coffee with him.

"Do you know what love is, mate?"

I look at him, he's wearing lunch-stained clothes and like all 'characters' has a colour to his skin that suggests he is carrying the town's grime with him.

I pull a non-committal face that suggests I'm not thinking of answering, but he continues.

"I can chart each of the loves of my life by their scent."

I'm worried he is going to share too much information and I look downwards and then out over the bar, hoping someone will to come to my aid.

"The first one; we were teenagers. She wore heavy floral scents, probably cheap. Well, she would have only been 16 when we met, no money you see. She'd have got the perfume off the indoor market and it would have had some ridiculous name. I reckon it was called something like Paris Love or Passion Flower Nights or something... I stayed with her for ten years and I remember, as we got a bit of money, she bought heavier scents, darker perfume, liquids in the bottle with more notes. You aware of the concept of 'notes' in perfume?" he asked.

I nodded.

"She left me for a plasterer. And then I fell in love with a sophisticated woman, expensive scent, chiffon scarfs and silk blouses... we didn't, you know, live together or anything, but I asked her the name of the perfume and she told me. I thought if I meet someone who wears that, she's the one for me... I never found one who was available though... all beyond me, I think.

The next one, the mother of my two boys; she had a very different scent. I always thought... she smelt of woods and berries, smelt of nature. But after 15 years I realised, these weren't natural smells at all. They were made in a laboratory somewhere and sold to women who wanted an earthy appeal. That was her all over, as fake a woman as you might meet."

He chuckled to himself.

"I couldn't stand the falseness, so I left. The boys don't speak to me now. I don't blame them. Then I met Janice. She had no smell, I held her in my arms at night and there was just her...nothing in the way... but she died and now there's just me and a head full of smells and memories. So what about you buddy?"

"Oh err, I haven't found anyone yet." I said.

"I've told women I love them, but that's because that's what they want to hear... they were just placeholders, until I find the love of my life."

He tapped my arm and looked into my eyes. I noticed that he had clear, bright, green-grey eyes.

"Look I'm just a simple man... can you explain to me... the difference between telling someone you love them and what you think you're going to find, when the real thing comes along?"

AN EDUCATION

1967. Britain is emerging from post war austerity into the brave consumerist world, allegedly.
A young boy is trailing a few feet behind his mother with his younger brother in a pram.

They walk past the big, three-storey, detached houses opposite the park. It is Saturday and men are fastidiously washing cars on their drives. The small family walk past the pretty two-storey semis in the bright sunshine. They pass the neat two-up two-down terraces with little front gardens fenced off and then head across wasteland that was previously allotments before the land was bought for development and the gardeners turfed off.

Next, they are walking down a street of derelict terraced houses with no front gardens. It is uncertain if they were inhabited, although the odd broken window gives away the fact that they are empty.

Then, in the middle of the row of houses, two houses have no windows at all, and one has no front door. The boy looks in and sees a flea bitten sofa and bare floorboards, although the floorboards have a sort of floor covering, namely pools coupons spread all over the room. For all the world the boy thinks that the previous incumbents must have won the pools and cast coupons all over the floor in their celebration. They have then moved on, he thinks, to a house far more luxurious than the three-storey detached houses opposite the park.

The boy decides that this must be what life and luck is all about... escaping the drudgery and misery of the grey streets by winning that precursor to today's National Lottery, The Pools, where for a few pence and eight crosses in the correct boxes, you can skip out of the door, not turn the lights off and join Viv Nicholson, who at that time had not spent, spent, spent.

The boy's mother knew that here had lived, Albert Quigley, who had been sentenced to 8 years for aggravated burglary and who had left Barbara Quigley with four children under ten. His mother did not tell deflate the boy's fantasy idea. Perhaps she should have done.

LITTLE GREEN LIGHT

In the month that my mum died, 100,000 fish were found dead in the Wutan province of China and 3.5 million birds died from a virus in Mexico. Mum always said she liked neither fish nor fowl. I thought at the time that this was Mum's form of extreme species eradication from the afterlife.

A couple of days after she died, I saw something shining bright on the road, near Sareth's house. It turned out to be a little green LED attached to a piece of plastic. The light shone even though it was disconnected from a power source of any description. I was very taken with this strange find and placed it on my car's dashboard.

When people got into the passenger seat, they would ask what it was. I would say, with as much mystery as I could muster, that it was my mum's soul and it was a comfort to me. I ignored the raised eyebrows and quizzical facial gestures. They could think what they liked.

In the days thereafter, I regularly checked the light, but still it shone. I lay in bed thinking that I must discover what the various religions think of the soul's migration into the afterlife and therefore see if they could predict how long this light would continue to shine.

This may all seem inappropriately whimsical, after what for me was real emotional grief as the loss of a mother would be to anyone. However, without properly verbalising it, I was genuinely comforted by the thought that my mum was there in the car with me whilst I drove.

So what was the reality? Could my ever-so combative mother have inhabited a little piece of electronic plastic, perhaps manufactured in an Asian sweatshop? Was I emotionally immature to be comforted in such a trite way? Should I have just thrown it out and dismissed this little diversion? Am I trying to make myself interesting in telling this story?

By the way, the light never went out.

SNAPSHOTS OF A STROKE RECOVERY

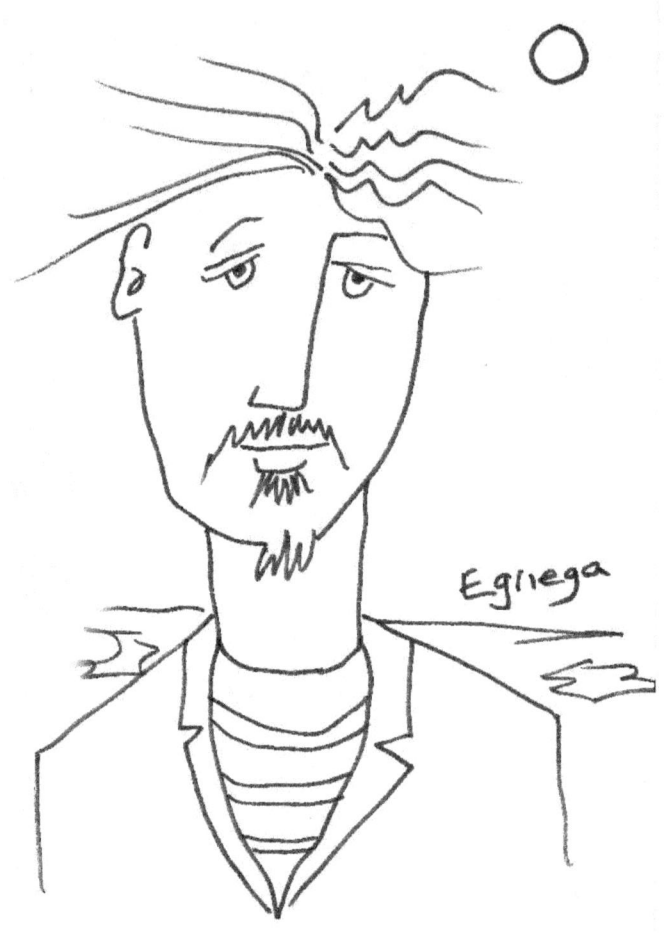

A SONG

All the umbrellas have been skiving and so the streets are soaking wet.
There's an orange girl and a paper boy, they don't know what they're going to get.
Reason makes them think that it's something that they'll want.
The world looks all right tonight.

The stars have been dazzling in the sky and on the ground.
They may be saying something, but they do not make a sound,
But if it is bad news, it will not bring me down.
The world looks all right tonight.

High up on the hillside, people looking down below.
They think they know it all but there's so much they don't know.
They've been riding their luck, but there's a long way to go.
The world looks all right tonight.

Take good care of my little one... switch the light off when she goes to sleep.
Please say a prayer for my little one, the world's a scary place when you're free.

My engine's shagged and my exhaust's shot and
my tyres are in a mess.
I haven't made much money... what the hell did I
expect?
But I'm lying in the dark and her arms they hold me
tight.
The world looks all right tonight.

ABOUT THE AUTHOR

Pieter Egriega had a first career as a guitarist in the late 70s and 80s as Arthur Kadmon. According to some sources he was described as 'the best talent who never made it'.

After his various 80s musical projects disbanded, he worked as a company director of a commercial business publishing company and supported a family. But then about four years ago he emerged as Pieter Egriega, tango singer-songwriter.

If you would like to write to Pieter, you can do so by e-mailing him at:
pieter@egriega.co.uk

To book Pieter for public speaking or musical performances:
management@egriega.co.uk

Learn more about Pieter by going to:
www.egriega.co.uk

PIETER EGRIEGA

STROKE

In the UK someone has a stroke every
three and half minutes.

Stroke is the third single largest cause of death
and the leading cause of adult disability in the UK.

Three in 10 stroke survivors will go on to have a
recurrent stroke or TIA (Transient Ischaemic
Attack).

There are around 1.2 million stroke survivors in
the UK.

For more information about stroke
ring the Helpline on 0303 3033 100 or visit
www.stroke.org.uk

PIETER EGRIEGA

www.ingramcontent.com/pod-product-compliance
Lightning Source LLC
Chambersburg PA
CBHW070356290526
45790CB00004B/1518